Manage Hypothyroidism Naturally

(5 Easy Steps)

A Practical Guide to Supporting Your Thyroid Health

By
Payal Patel

Introduction

Hypothyroidism is a complex condition characterized by the underproduction of thyroid hormones by the thyroid gland, a small butterfly-shaped gland located in the front of the neck. This gland plays a critical role in regulating various bodily functions, including metabolism, energy production, heart rate, and even mood regulation. When the thyroid is underactive, it can lead to an array of symptoms that significantly impact an individual's daily life. These symptoms may include persistent fatigue that can make even simple tasks feel overwhelming, unintentional weight gain despite normal eating habits, hair thinning or loss, dry skin, and cognitive challenges like memory lapses, brain fog, and difficulty concentrating. As these symptoms manifest, they often lead to frustration and feelings of helplessness, affecting overall quality of life.

For many individuals diagnosed with hypothyroidism, conventional treatments typically involve prescribed medications such as levothyroxine, which aims to replace the missing thyroid hormones. However, for some, these medications may not provide the desired relief or can lead to side effects, such as anxiety, insomnia, or digestive issues. This experience can leave individuals feeling trapped in a cycle of ineffective treatment, leading to hopelessness and a desperate search for answers.

Recognizing the limitations of traditional treatments, a growing number of people are seeking alternative and complementary approaches to manage their hypothyroidism. This guide delves into effective natural methods to support thyroid health and enhance well-being. We will explore practical lifestyle changes, including dietary adjustments that prioritize nutrient-dense foods rich in vitamins and minerals essential for thyroid function, as well as the incorporation of regular physical activity to boost metabolism and energy levels. Stress management techniques, such as mindfulness practices and relaxation exercises, are also emphasized, as stress can exacerbate thyroid symptoms.

Additionally, we will discuss the importance of proper supplementation, including whole-food multivitamins and targeted nutrients that support thyroid function and overall health. By focusing on these holistic strategies, you can empower yourself to take charge of your health and navigate your hypothyroidism more effectively. This guide aims to provide you with the knowledge and tools necessary to reclaim your vitality and enhance your quality of life while managing hypothyroidism naturally.

Understanding Hypothyroidism

Hypothyroidism is a condition that arises when the thyroid gland, a small but crucial organ located at the base of the neck, becomes underactive. This underactivity results in insufficient production of thyroid hormones, which are essential for regulating numerous bodily functions, including metabolism, heart rate, temperature control, and even mood stability. The thyroid hormones—primarily thyroxine (T4) and triiodothyronine (T3)—are vital in maintaining the body's energy levels and overall health. When hormone levels drop, the body can experience a cascade of physiological changes that significantly affect well-being.

The causes of hypothyroidism can be diverse and multifaceted. One of the most common causes is autoimmune disorders, particularly Hashimoto's thyroiditis, where the immune system mistakenly attacks the thyroid gland, leading to inflammation and impaired hormone production. Additionally, certain medications, such as lithium and some treatments for hyperthyroidism, can contribute to the development of hypothyroidism. Nutritional deficiencies, especially of iodine, selenium, and zinc, can also play a critical role in thyroid health, as these nutrients are essential for hormone synthesis and metabolism. Identifying these underlying factors is crucial for understanding the condition and effectively managing it.

Recognizing the symptoms of hypothyroidism is essential for those who suspect they may be affected. Common symptoms include:

- **Fatigue**: One of the hallmark symptoms, fatigue in hypothyroidism can feel like an overwhelming sense of tiredness that persists despite adequate sleep. Many individuals report waking up in the morning feeling as if they haven't rested at all, making it challenging to engage in daily activities or maintain productivity.
- **Weight Gain**: Unexplained weight gain can be particularly disheartening for those with hypothyroidism. Despite efforts in diet and exercise, many find themselves gaining weight, leading to feelings of frustration and disappointment as they struggle to achieve their health goals.
- **Cold Intolerance**: Individuals with hypothyroidism often experience cold intolerance, a constant chill that makes them feel uncomfortable in environments where others may feel perfectly fine. This sensitivity can extend to cooler temperatures and can significantly affect daily life and social activities.
- **Depression and Anxiety**: The emotional toll of hypothyroidism can manifest as depression and

anxiety. These emotional lows can feel isolating, as though a dark cloud is following you around. Individuals may experience mood swings, irritability, and a general sense of hopelessness, compounding the physical symptoms they are already facing.

- **Cognitive Issues**: Cognitive impairment, often described as "brain fog," can make daily life increasingly challenging. Individuals may struggle with concentration, experience forgetfulness, and find it difficult to process information. This cognitive decline can impact both personal and professional productivity, leading to frustration and a decrease in quality of life.

Understanding these symptoms is crucial for recognizing how hypothyroidism can impact your life. By being aware of the signs, individuals can seek medical advice, undergo appropriate testing, and pursue effective solutions tailored to their unique needs. This knowledge empowers those affected to take proactive steps toward managing their health and reclaiming their well-being.

My Personal Journey

My journey with hypothyroidism began several years ago, and it feels like a chapter from a book I never wanted to write. It started subtly, almost imperceptibly, as a creeping fatigue that seemed to seep into my very bones. No matter how much sleep I got, I would wake up feeling as if I had run a marathon the day before, my body heavy and unwilling to move. I remember those mornings vividly—sitting on the edge of my bed, battling the overwhelming sensation that I had not rested at all. As the days turned into weeks, I began to notice something even more alarming: despite my efforts to eat healthily and stay active, the scale tipped higher. Each increase in weight felt like another layer of defeat, deepening my frustration and disillusionment.

The emotional toll of these changes was profound. I felt defeated, frustrated, and isolated, as if I were the only person in the world struggling with an invisible burden. It seemed like no matter how hard I tried, my body was betraying me. Simple tasks became monumental challenges, and I often found myself withdrawing from social situations, fearing I would be unable to keep up. After numerous doctor visits and a seemingly endless cycle of blood tests, I finally received a diagnosis: hypothyroidism. My doctor prescribed medication, and while I hoped for relief, I continued to grapple with the same relentless symptoms. The medications provided some relief but were not the miracle cure I had desperately sought. I still felt a cloud of fatigue hovering over me, casting a shadow over my daily life.

Desperate for change and determined to reclaim my life, I embarked on a quest for natural remedies. It was during this search that I stumbled upon Ayurveda, an ancient Indian healing system that emphasizes balance within the body through lifestyle and dietary adjustments. The idea of managing my condition holistically resonated deeply with me, igniting a flicker of hope I hadn't felt in a long time. I was drawn to the principles of Ayurveda, which advocates for individualized care and encourages a connection to nature and self.

I committed to embracing an Ayurvedic lifestyle, which included adopting a nutrient-rich diet filled with whole foods and vibrant colors. I began practicing intermittent fasting, initially facing the challenges of hunger pangs that tested my resolve. However, as the days passed, I slowly began to feel lighter and more energized, a welcome contrast to the heaviness I had been carrying. I vividly remember the first time I prepared a meal that celebrated my health—each ingredient was chosen with care, each color a reminder of the nourishment I was providing my body. Cooking transformed into a joyful ritual, a mindful act of self-care that deepened my appreciation for food.

As I made these changes, I discovered the profound connection between what I ate and how I felt. With each passing day, my energy levels began to improve, my mood stabilized, and I started to feel like myself again. This journey taught me invaluable lessons in resilience and self-advocacy. I learned to listen to my body and trust its signals, a skill that felt both empowering and liberating.

Now, I feel equipped with the tools to manage my condition naturally, and I share my story not just to inform but to inspire anyone facing similar challenges. My hope is that others will explore natural solutions that resonate with them, understanding that they, too, have the power to reclaim their health and well-being. This journey has transformed my life, and I believe it can do the same for others who feel lost in their struggle with hypothyroidism.

Step 1: Optimize Your Diet

Healthy Diet

A balanced, nutrient-rich diet is essential for effectively managing hypothyroidism and supporting overall health. Your dietary choices can have a profound impact on thyroid function, energy levels, and emotional well-being. To cultivate a diet that nourishes your body and promotes thyroid health, focus on incorporating a wide variety of whole, unprocessed foods that are rich in essential vitamins and minerals.

Start by integrating leafy greens such as spinach, kale, and Swiss chard into your meals. These nutrient-dense vegetables are high in antioxidants and provide vital nutrients that can help protect your thyroid gland from oxidative stress. Additionally, nuts and seeds like walnuts, flaxseeds, and chia seeds are excellent sources of omega-3 fatty acids, which possess anti-inflammatory properties that can support thyroid function and overall hormone balance.

Whole grains should also be a staple in your diet, as they provide essential fiber, vitamins, and minerals. Quinoa, brown rice, and oats not only promote digestive health but also contribute to sustained energy levels throughout the day.

Additionally, foods rich in selenium, such as Brazil nuts, play a crucial role in the conversion of T4 to T3, the active form of thyroid hormone. A small handful of Brazil nuts can provide you with an adequate daily dose of this essential nutrient.

Zinc-rich foods, such as chickpeas, lentils, and pumpkin seeds, are vital for maintaining healthy thyroid function and hormone production. Zinc supports the synthesis of thyroid hormones and helps the body utilize them effectively. Including these foods in your meals can be as simple as adding chickpeas to salads or soups or snacking on pumpkin seeds throughout the day.

Iodine is another critical nutrient for thyroid health, as it is essential for the production of thyroid hormones. Sources of iodine include seaweed, such as nori and kelp, which can be easily incorporated into your diet. Whether in the form of sushi, salads, or soups, seaweed adds a savory flavor while boosting your iodine levels.

While focusing on nutrient-rich foods, it is equally important to be mindful of what to avoid. Processed foods, which often contain additives, unhealthy fats, and sugars, can interfere with thyroid hormone production and lead to inflammation. Steer clear of these foods whenever possible and opt for fresh, whole ingredients instead.

Some foods can hinder thyroid function, particularly in sensitive individuals. Soy products, such as tofu and soy milk, contain phytoestrogens that can disrupt hormone balance, especially when consumed in large quantities. Cruciferous vegetables, including broccoli, cauliflower, and Brussels sprouts, are healthy when cooked but can interfere with iodine uptake when consumed raw in excessive amounts. If you love these vegetables, consider steaming or roasting them to reduce their goitrogenic effects.

Additionally, many people with thyroid conditions may find it beneficial to limit gluten in their diets, particularly if they have gluten sensitivity or celiac disease. This can help alleviate any additional stress on the immune system and reduce inflammation.

Don't forget to include healthy fats in your diet. Sources such as avocados, olive oil, and nuts provide the essential fatty acids your body needs for hormone production and overall well-being. Healthy fats support brain function, improve nutrient absorption, and help maintain stable energy levels, making them an essential component of a thyroid-friendly diet.

In summary, a healthy diet for managing hypothyroidism involves embracing a variety of nutrient-dense, whole foods while avoiding those that can hinder thyroid function. By prioritizing foods that support thyroid health and nurturing your body with balanced nutrition, you can take significant strides toward improving your energy levels, mood, and overall well-being.

Intermittent Fasting

Intermittent fasting (IF) has emerged as a powerful tool for managing various health conditions, including hypothyroidism. At its core, intermittent fasting involves cycling between periods of eating and fasting, allowing your body to undergo various beneficial processes during the fasting phase. One of the most popular methods is the 16:8 approach, where you fast for 16 hours and limit your eating to an 8-hour window each day. This method not only simplifies meal planning but also promotes a range of health benefits that can significantly improve your overall well-being.

During the fasting period, your digestive system gets a much-needed break. This rest allows your body to redirect its energy toward vital repair and rejuvenation processes, such as detoxification and cellular regeneration. When you fast, insulin levels drop, which can enhance fat metabolism and improve your body's ability to burn stored fat for energy. For individuals with hypothyroidism, weight management can be a persistent struggle, and intermittent fasting may provide a practical solution by promoting metabolic efficiency.

Additionally, intermittent fasting can positively influence hormonal balance. As your body enters a fasting state, levels of human growth hormone (HGH) can increase significantly, enhancing muscle mass and promoting fat loss. The reduction in insulin levels also allows for better regulation of other hormones that are critical for thyroid function. By optimizing hormone levels, intermittent fasting can help alleviate some of the symptoms associated with hypothyroidism, such as fatigue and weight gain.

It's important, however, to approach intermittent fasting with caution, especially if you are new to it. Start gradually, perhaps by shortening your eating window or skipping one meal a few times a week. This gentle approach allows your body to adjust without overwhelming your system. Pay attention to how your body responds; it's essential to listen to your hunger cues and energy levels. If you find yourself feeling excessively fatigued or irritable, it might be a sign to ease up on your fasting regimen.

During your eating window, prioritize nutrient-dense meals that support your thyroid health and overall vitality. Focus on incorporating whole foods rich in vitamins, minerals, and healthy fats. Meals should be well-balanced and satisfying, including an array of colorful vegetables, lean proteins, whole grains, and healthy fats. This nutritional approach will help maintain stable energy levels throughout the day, allowing you to reap the benefits of intermittent fasting without sacrificing your well-being.

As you adapt to intermittent fasting, you may begin to notice subtle shifts in your energy levels and overall mood. Many individuals report enhanced mental clarity, increased focus, and improved resilience against fatigue during their fasting periods. This clarity can be especially beneficial for those struggling with cognitive issues associated with hypothyroidism. Furthermore, intermittent fasting may promote better sleep quality, which is crucial for hormone regulation and overall health.

In summary, intermittent fasting can be a valuable strategy for managing hypothyroidism by promoting digestive rest, improving metabolic function, and supporting hormonal balance. By embracing this eating pattern mindfully and focusing on nutrient-rich meals, you can harness the benefits of intermittent fasting while nurturing your thyroid health and enhancing your overall quality of life. As with any dietary change, it's essential to consult with a healthcare professional before starting intermittent fasting, especially if you have specific health concerns related to your thyroid condition.

Foods to Include

Iodine-Rich Foods

Iodine is a key mineral when it comes to thyroid health, as it plays a central role in the production of thyroid hormones. Without sufficient iodine, your thyroid cannot produce enough of the hormones that regulate metabolism, energy levels, and overall well-being. For those managing hypothyroidism, including iodine-rich foods in your diet is essential to support thyroid function. Some of the best natural sources of iodine include seaweed, fish, and eggs.

Seaweed, such as nori, kelp, and wakame, is an incredibly potent source of iodine. In fact, a single serving of seaweed can often provide more than the recommended daily intake of iodine. I still remember the first time I tried seaweed snacks; the salty, slightly briny crunch was a delightful change from my usual snacks. At first, the unique flavor took a bit of getting used to, but over time I came to appreciate the rich taste and the knowledge that I was actively nourishing my thyroid. It became a satisfying, guilt-free snack that I could enjoy while feeling proud of making a health-conscious choice.

Fish, especially cold-water varieties like salmon, tuna, and cod, are also excellent sources of iodine and omega-3 fatty acids, which support both thyroid and heart health. Incorporating fish into my meals was a simple but effective way to boost my iodine intake while also reaping the benefits of healthy fats. The versatility of fish allowed me to experiment with different recipes—baked salmon with lemon and herbs became a weekly favorite, filling my kitchen with comforting aromas while providing my body with the nutrients it craved.

Eggs are another readily accessible source of iodine, particularly found in the yolk. Including eggs in my breakfast routine not only helped support my thyroid but also kept me feeling full and energized throughout the day. Whether scrambled, poached, or added to a vibrant vegetable stir-fry, eggs became a quick, easy, and delicious way to nourish my thyroid each morning.

Selenium

Selenium is another crucial mineral that plays an integral role in thyroid health. It helps protect the thyroid from oxidative stress and is necessary for converting the inactive thyroid hormone (T4) into its active form (T3), which the body can use.

Without enough selenium, thyroid function can become impaired, leading to worsened symptoms of hypothyroidism. Fortunately, selenium is easy to incorporate into your diet through foods such as Brazil nuts, sunflower seeds, and legumes.

I discovered the power of Brazil nuts when I started researching selenium-rich foods. Just two Brazil nuts a day can provide your entire daily requirement of selenium. They became a staple snack for me—simple, convenient, and packed with health benefits. I even kept a jar of them on my desk at work, and each time I reached for a handful, I felt a sense of accomplishment knowing I was giving my thyroid the support it needed. The crunchy texture and slightly creamy taste were bonuses that made this healthy habit easy to maintain.

Sunflower seeds are another selenium-rich food that I often sprinkled on salads or added to smoothies. Their mild flavor and crunchy texture made them a versatile addition to my meals, and they provided a satisfying boost of nutrients, particularly when I was feeling low on energy. On busy days, a handful of sunflower seeds would tide me over, keeping my energy levels steady without relying on processed snacks.

For variety, I also embraced legumes like lentils, chickpeas, and black beans. Not only are they rich in selenium, but they also offer plant-based protein and fiber, which helps regulate digestion and keeps me feeling full for longer. I found that adding legumes to soups, salads, and stews was a great way to increase my selenium intake while enjoying hearty, satisfying meals. Over time, I noticed a gradual improvement in my energy levels and overall mood as my body responded to the increased intake of selenium.

Anti-Inflammatory Foods

Incorporating anti-inflammatory foods into your diet is key to managing hypothyroidism, as inflammation can exacerbate thyroid dysfunction and contribute to symptoms like fatigue, brain fog, and mood swings. These foods, particularly colorful fruits and vegetables, help reduce inflammation in the body and provide a wealth of antioxidants and vitamins that support overall health. I began prioritizing foods like leafy greens, berries, and turmeric to create meals that were as vibrant as they were nutritious.

One of my favorite routines became preparing a vibrant salad filled with anti-inflammatory ingredients, such as spinach, arugula, and kale. Topped with antioxidant-rich berries like blueberries and raspberries, and drizzled with olive oil and lemon, each salad felt like a celebration of color and health. The process of chopping and arranging the ingredients became a mindful act of self-care, and the flavors—sweet, tangy, and fresh—were a reminder that healthy eating could be truly enjoyable.

I also discovered the profound benefits of turmeric, an anti-inflammatory spice that has been used in Ayurvedic medicine for centuries. Adding a teaspoon of turmeric to soups, curries, or even smoothies became a daily habit. I especially loved making turmeric lattes, blending the golden spice with almond milk, cinnamon, and a touch of honey. This soothing drink not only helped reduce inflammation but also brought a sense of warmth and comfort, particularly on chilly days.

Eating these anti-inflammatory foods regularly became a cornerstone of my healing journey. As I focused on adding these vibrant, nutrient-dense ingredients to my diet, I noticed significant improvements in how I felt—less brain fog, more energy, and a calmer, more stable mood. Each meal became an opportunity to nourish my body from the inside out, and over time, I began to feel more connected to my health and well-being.

Foods to Avoid

Goitrogens

Goitrogens are compounds found in certain foods that can interfere with thyroid function by inhibiting the uptake of iodine, which is essential for thyroid hormone production. While goitrogenic foods are generally nutritious and can be part of a healthy diet, consuming them in excessive amounts, especially raw, can impact those with hypothyroidism. Cruciferous vegetables such as broccoli, cauliflower, kale, Brussels sprouts, and cabbage are known goitrogenic foods, as well as soy products like tofu and soy milk.

When I first learned about the potential effects of goitrogens, I was disappointed. I loved eating kale salads and often snacked on raw broccoli. But after doing my research, I realized that I didn't have to eliminate these foods entirely—I just had to be mindful of how I prepared them. Cooking cruciferous vegetables lightly, such as steaming, blanching, or sautéing, helps to reduce their goitrogenic properties while retaining much of their nutritional value. I began incorporating lightly cooked greens into my meals instead of raw versions. For example, I would steam broccoli and toss it with garlic and olive oil, creating a dish that was both flavorful and thyroid-friendly.

Soy was another challenge. I had been using soy milk in my smoothies and loved adding tofu to stir-fries. After learning about its potential to affect thyroid function, I became more cautious about how often I included it in my diet. I didn't cut it out completely, but I made an effort to reduce my soy intake and replace it with alternatives like almond milk and tempeh in moderation. This small adjustment helped me feel more in control of my thyroid health without sacrificing variety in my diet.

Processed Foods

Processed foods are another major factor that can exacerbate symptoms of hypothyroidism. These foods are often high in unhealthy fats, refined sugars, and artificial additives, all of which can lead to inflammation and wreak havoc on your metabolism. The convenience of processed snacks like chips, cookies, and packaged meals often comes at the expense of long-term health.

In my journey toward healing, I made a conscious effort to eliminate processed foods from my diet. Initially, it was challenging—like many people, I relied on quick snacks to get through busy days. But as I became more aware of how these foods impacted my body, I realized that the short-term satisfaction wasn't worth the long-term fatigue and sluggishness I felt afterward.

I started to experiment with homemade alternatives, creating simple, healthy snacks that were easy to grab on the go. I began making energy balls from oats, nuts, and dates, as well as homemade granola with nuts and seeds. These snacks were not only delicious but also packed with the nutrients my body needed to support thyroid health. The difference in how I felt was remarkable—my energy levels became more consistent throughout the day, and I no longer experienced the sugar crashes that often followed processed snacks.

Another aspect I focused on was preparing my meals ahead of time to avoid relying on packaged foods. I began batch-cooking whole grain salads, vegetable soups, and quinoa bowls, which I could quickly heat up when I needed a nourishing meal. Over time, this shift toward whole, minimally processed foods helped reduce inflammation and improved my overall well-being.

Gluten

For many people with hypothyroidism, particularly those with Hashimoto's thyroiditis, gluten can be a significant trigger for inflammation and worsened symptoms. Gluten, a protein found in wheat, barley, and rye, can sometimes cause an immune response in the body that affects the thyroid. Because of this, some people with thyroid issues find that eliminating gluten from their diet helps alleviate symptoms like fatigue, bloating, and brain fog.

At first, I was hesitant to try eliminating gluten. I had grown up eating gluten-rich foods like wheat roti, pasta, and bread, and the idea of cutting them out felt daunting. But after experiencing persistent symptoms despite my medication and dietary adjustments, I decided to give a gluten-free diet a try. The first few weeks were challenging—I had to rethink many of my usual meals and find alternatives to my favorite breads and pastas. But as I ventured into the world of gluten-free grains like quinoa, brown rice, and millet, I discovered that there were plenty of delicious options available.

I remember the first time I made a gluten-free quinoa and chickpea salad—it was filling, flavorful, and surprisingly satisfying. I began experimenting with more recipes, like gluten-free oat pancakes and buckwheat soba noodles, which opened my eyes to new flavors and textures. Slowly but surely, my cravings for gluten subsided, and I noticed improvements in my digestion and energy levels.

Though not everyone with hypothyroidism needs to eliminate gluten, I found that this dietary change made a noticeable difference in my health. It wasn't just about giving up gluten; it was about discovering new ways to nourish my body and creating meals that aligned with my health goals. The experience taught me that sometimes, the foods we rely on most can be the ones holding us back, and making mindful adjustments can lead to profound changes in how we feel.

Step 2: Incorporate Regular Exercise

Aerobic Exercise

Aerobic exercise, often referred to as "cardio," is essential for boosting metabolism and improving overall cardiovascular health. Activities like walking, jogging, cycling, and even swimming fall under this category. For those with hypothyroidism, aerobic exercise can also help combat the sluggish metabolism that often accompanies the condition, promoting better energy utilization and fat burning.

When I first started incorporating aerobic exercise, I opted for simple, low-impact activities. I began with brisk walks, enjoying the crisp morning air and the quiet moments to myself. Initially, I could barely keep up a fast pace for more than 10 minutes, but as the days went by, my stamina gradually increased. The fresh air, combined with the rhythm of my steps, helped me clear my mind and gave me a renewed sense of purpose each day. Eventually, I worked my way up to light jogging, feeling more empowered as my endurance improved.

One of the most surprising benefits was the mental clarity I experienced after these walks. On days when my thyroid symptoms made me feel foggy and tired, even a short 20-minute walk was enough to lift my spirits and reenergize me. I learned to rely on these aerobic sessions as both a physical and mental reset.

Strength Training

Strength training is an often-overlooked but incredibly important component of exercise for those with hypothyroidism. When muscle mass increases, so does the resting metabolic rate—meaning you burn more calories even when you're not actively working out. This is especially beneficial for those who struggle with weight management due to a sluggish metabolism.

I was initially intimidated by the idea of lifting weights, but I soon realized that strength training didn't have to involve heavy dumbbells or complex gym equipment. I started with bodyweight exercises like push-ups, squats, and lunges, as well as simple resistance bands that I could use at home. These exercises required minimal equipment but provided maximum benefits. I could feel myself getting stronger with each session, and the improvement in my physical strength had a direct impact on my confidence and mood.

Strength training also gave me a sense of empowerment. The ability to lift more, move more fluidly, and feel physically capable improved my overall outlook. I enjoyed how my muscles felt more toned, and over time, I noticed a difference in how my body responded to other forms of exercise.

Flexibility Exercises

Flexibility exercises like yoga, stretching, or Pilates play a key role in overall well-being, especially for people managing hypothyroidism. These exercises not only enhance physical flexibility but also contribute to stress reduction, which is critical for thyroid health. Chronic stress can interfere with hormone production and exacerbate symptoms, so managing stress through mindful movement can have a profound effect.

I started attending a local yoga class once a week, and it quickly became a highlight in my schedule. The gentle stretches, combined with deep breathing techniques, helped me release tension I didn't even realize I was holding. The physical benefits were clear—I became more flexible and balanced—but the mental clarity and relaxation I gained from each session were equally transformative.

Yoga helped me create a mind-body connection that I had not explored before. Each pose allowed me to focus inward, reducing the anxiety and stress I often felt due to my thyroid condition. It wasn't just about the exercise; it was about reclaiming a sense of control over my body and mind. Even simple stretching routines in the morning or before bed became a way for me to relax and check in with myself, noticing where I was holding stress and releasing it consciously.

Benefits of Physical Activity

The benefits of regular physical activity extend far beyond weight management. While it's true that exercise helps boost metabolism, what stood out most for me was the impact on my mood, energy levels, and cognitive function. One of the most frustrating symptoms of hypothyroidism is brain fog—a feeling of mental sluggishness that can make even simple tasks feel daunting. I noticed that after just a short workout, my mind felt clearer, and I was able to focus better on my work and daily tasks.

Exercise also helped combat the fatigue that seemed to linger no matter how much rest I got. On days when I felt particularly tired, I would push myself to complete even a 15-minute session of walking or strength training, and almost every time, I felt more energized afterward. The endorphins released during exercise gave me a natural boost, making it easier to stay positive and focused throughout the day.

Moreover, physical activity became a crucial tool in helping me manage my emotional health. The connection between thyroid function and mood swings can be difficult to navigate, but regular exercise helped me maintain a sense of balance. It reduced my feelings of anxiety and depression, allowing me to feel more grounded and resilient in the face of challenges. Over time, I began to view exercise not as a chore, but as a form of self-care, an investment in both my physical and emotional well-being.

Through aerobic exercise, strength training, and flexibility exercises, I built a routine that not only supported my thyroid health but also became a vital part of my life. These practices empowered me to feel stronger, more capable, and more in control of my body and my health journey.

Step 3: Manage Stress Effectively

Stress Reduction Techniques

Yoga

Yoga is an ancient practice that combines physical postures (asanas), breathing exercises (pranayama), and meditation to create a holistic approach to stress reduction. For those with hypothyroidism, yoga not only offers physical benefits, such as improving flexibility and circulation, but it also plays a crucial role in reducing stress—a significant factor that can exacerbate thyroid issues. The interplay of mind and body in yoga promotes a state of calm and balance, which can help regulate hormonal fluctuations.

When I first began practicing yoga, it became more than just exercise; it became a sanctuary. Each time I stepped onto my mat, I felt like I was entering a space where I could release the worries of the day. I focused on gentle movements that stretched my body without causing strain. The practice of holding poses while focusing on my breath helped me connect with my body in a way I hadn't before. Poses like Child's Pose and Legs-Up-the-Wall became my go-to for moments of deep relaxation. These postures, combined with slow, deep breaths, allowed me to access a sense of peace that I had been missing, especially during periods of heightened stress and fatigue.

Yoga also helped me cultivate mental clarity. The act of focusing on my breath and movements provided a form of active meditation, helping me let go of racing thoughts and anxiety. I started attending classes regularly, and it became something I truly looked forward to—a time carved out just for me. Over time, I noticed a shift in how I responded to stress. Instead of feeling overwhelmed, I could approach challenges with more composure, largely thanks to the grounding effects of yoga.

Meditation

Meditation is a powerful tool for managing both mental and emotional stress, particularly for individuals living with hypothyroidism. The practice of mindfulness meditation involves focusing on the present moment without judgment, which can help calm the mind and reduce cortisol levels—a stress hormone that can interfere with thyroid function. For many, hypothyroidism brings about feelings of anxiety and frustration, and meditation offers a way to regain control over these emotions.

I started meditating by dedicating just five minutes a day to sitting quietly, focusing on my breath. Initially, my mind would wander, and I found it hard to stay present. But with consistency, I began to notice a shift. Those five minutes became a sacred pause in my day, where I could slow down and simply be. The more I practiced, the better I became at noticing when I was getting caught up in negative thought patterns, allowing me to gently bring my attention back to my breath. Eventually, I extended my practice to ten or twenty minutes, and I found that it made a world of difference in my ability to handle stress.

Meditation gave me a sense of emotional regulation. In moments of high stress, I could tap into the calm I had cultivated during my sessions, allowing me to approach situations with more patience and perspective. This ability to remain centered amidst chaos was a profound gift, especially as I navigated the ups and downs of managing my thyroid condition.

Deep-Breathing Exercises

Deep-breathing exercises are a simple yet incredibly effective way to quickly reduce stress and promote relaxation. Diaphragmatic breathing, also known as belly breathing, helps stimulate the parasympathetic nervous system, which is responsible for calming the body. For individuals with hypothyroidism, managing stress is crucial to supporting thyroid health, as chronic stress can exacerbate symptoms like fatigue and brain fog.

I began incorporating deep-breathing exercises into my daily routine, particularly during moments of overwhelm. Whenever I felt tension building up—whether from work, family responsibilities, or just the weight of daily life—I would take a moment to pause and focus on my breath. I started with the simple technique of inhaling deeply through my nose for four counts, holding for four counts, and then exhaling slowly through my mouth for another four counts. This small, intentional action would immediately help release the tightness in my chest and shoulders.

Over time, I began using these breathing exercises as a preventive measure, practicing them first thing in the morning to set a calm tone for the day, and then again before bed to wind down. The beauty of deep-breathing exercises is that they can be done anywhere, anytime—in the car, at your desk, or even while waiting in line. It became my go-to tool for navigating stressful situations, giving me a sense of control over my body's response to external pressures.

Mindfulness and Relaxation Practices

Mindfulness is the practice of being fully present in the moment, observing thoughts and feelings without judgment. For those managing hypothyroidism, integrating mindfulness into daily life can help reduce the impact of stress on both the mind and body. Stress can lead to a cascade of negative effects, including hormonal imbalances that further impair thyroid function. By practicing mindfulness, I found a way to create moments of calm amidst the busyness of life, which helped me manage my thyroid symptoms more effectively.

At first, I thought mindfulness was just another term for meditation, but I quickly learned that it could be practiced in small, intentional ways throughout the day. I began by dedicating a few minutes each morning to sit quietly, breathe, and simply observe my thoughts without reacting to them. This daily ritual fostered a sense of self-awareness that carried into the rest of my day. When stressful moments arose, I was better equipped to pause, breathe, and respond thoughtfully rather than react out of frustration.

Mindfulness also became a part of my everyday activities. Whether I was cooking, walking, or even folding laundry, I practiced being fully engaged in the moment—paying attention to the sounds, smells, and textures around me. These simple acts of presence helped me feel more grounded and reduced the constant mental chatter that often led to stress. In moments where I felt overwhelmed, taking just a few mindful breaths helped me reset, bringing a sense of calm and balance to my day.

By incorporating stress-reduction techniques like yoga, meditation, deep-breathing exercises, and mindfulness into my routine, I found not only physical relief but also emotional resilience. These practices have become a cornerstone of my approach to managing hypothyroidism naturally, providing me with tools to handle the stressors that used to feel overwhelming. Through these practices, I discovered that taking time to care for my mental and emotional well-being was just as important as focusing on my physical health.

Step 4: Monitor Your Supplements

Essential Vitamins and Minerals

Vitamin D: Crucial for Immune Function and Hormone Regulation

Vitamin D plays a key role in immune health and hormone balance, both of which are essential for managing hypothyroidism. Vitamin D helps regulate the immune system, reducing inflammation and supporting overall thyroid function. For those with hypothyroidism, low vitamin D levels are common, and addressing this deficiency can make a significant difference in symptom management.

When I first began to take my thyroid health seriously, I had my Vitamin D levels checked and discovered they were much lower than recommended. This came as no surprise, especially since I live in an area where sunlight is limited during the colder months. I started supplementing with Vitamin D3, and within weeks, I noticed improvements in my mood and energy levels. I also made an effort to spend more time outdoors when possible, allowing natural sunlight to help boost my vitamin D levels. Prioritizing this simple yet vital nutrient helped me feel more energized, especially during the winter months when my energy typically dipped.

B Vitamins: Vital for Energy Metabolism

The B vitamins, including B12, B6, and folate, are essential for energy production and help alleviate the fatigue that often accompanies hypothyroidism. These vitamins play a crucial role in supporting the nervous system and promoting proper brain function, both of which are often impacted by thyroid imbalances.

To address this, I made a conscious effort to include more B-vitamin-rich foods in my diet. Leafy greens like spinach and kale, quinoa, and legumes became regular staples in my meals. Incorporating these foods into my daily routine not only provided me with the necessary B vitamins but also gave me a sense of control over my health. Each meal felt like an opportunity to nourish my body and give it the tools it needed to thrive. Over time, I noticed that my fatigue started to lessen, and I could get through the day without feeling drained. The increase in energy levels was gradual but noticeable, giving me the encouragement to continue prioritizing these nutrients.

Zinc and Omega-3 Fatty Acids: Supporting Immune Health and Reducing Inflammation

Both zinc and omega-3 fatty acids are incredibly beneficial for thyroid health due to their anti-inflammatory properties and their ability to support the immune system. Zinc plays a direct role in thyroid hormone production, while omega-3s help reduce inflammation, which is especially important for those with autoimmune thyroid conditions like Hashimoto's disease.

To ensure I was getting enough of these essential nutrients, I added omega-3 supplements into my daily regimen, alongside foods like chia seeds and flaxseeds, which are plant-based sources of omega-3s. Not only did I feel the benefits in my thyroid health, but I also noticed a significant improvement in my skin and hair, which had suffered due to my hypothyroidism. The dry, brittle hair and flaky skin became more manageable, and I began to feel more confident in my appearance. Additionally, incorporating zinc-rich foods like chickpeas, nuts, and seeds gave my immune system a noticeable boost, especially during flu season. I felt more resilient and experienced fewer colds and infections compared to previous years.

Whole Food Multivitamin: Filling Nutrient Gaps

Even with a nutrient-rich diet, it can sometimes be difficult to meet all your body's needs, especially when managing a condition like hypothyroidism. To ensure I was consistently getting all the necessary vitamins and minerals for thyroid health, I began taking a whole-food multivitamin. Unlike synthetic supplements, whole-food vitamins are derived from natural sources and are more easily absorbed by the body, ensuring I was getting optimal nourishment.

Adding this multivitamin to my daily routine became a safety net, filling any potential nutrient gaps. It brought me peace of mind knowing that my thyroid was receiving the support it needed. Over time, I noticed a gradual improvement in my energy and mental clarity, which I attributed to the consistent intake of essential nutrients. This was particularly helpful during busy days when I didn't have the time to prepare nutrient-dense meals.

Liver Detox: Supporting Hormone Metabolism

The liver plays a critical role in hormone metabolism, including the conversion of thyroid hormones into their active form. A healthy liver ensures that thyroid hormones are processed efficiently, which is crucial for maintaining proper energy levels and overall well-being. Supporting liver health is particularly important for those with hypothyroidism, as the liver can become sluggish due to the metabolic challenges posed by the condition.

I began incorporating liver-friendly foods like beets, garlic, and dandelion root tea into my diet. These foods are known to support the liver's natural detoxification processes, helping it function optimally. I also took breaks from processed foods and alcohol, giving my liver time to recover and detoxify. This, combined with regular consumption of fiber-rich vegetables, helped improve my digestion and overall sense of well-being. I noticed that when my liver was functioning well, I felt lighter and more energized. This simple yet effective detoxification routine became a key part of my thyroid management plan, ensuring that my hormones were in balance and working as they should.

Herbal Remedies

Ashwagandha and Guggul: Ayurvedic Support for Thyroid Health

Ayurveda, the ancient system of Indian medicine, offers a wealth of herbal remedies that can help balance thyroid function and support overall health. Two herbs that have been particularly beneficial for managing hypothyroidism are ashwagandha and guggul. Ashwagandha is an adaptogen, meaning it helps the body cope with stress, which can be a major trigger for thyroid imbalances. It also supports the production of thyroid hormones and helps regulate the body's metabolism.

I started incorporating ashwagandha into my daily routine, either in the form of a supplement or as a powder added to my morning smoothies. Over time, I felt a noticeable improvement in my stress levels and mental clarity. The constant feeling of overwhelm that often accompanied my hypothyroidism began to diminish, and I felt more centered and in control of my emotions. The calming effects of ashwagandha also helped improve my sleep, which had been disrupted by thyroid imbalances.

In addition to ashwagandha, I explored the use of guggul, another herb known for its thyroid-supporting properties. Guggul helps to stimulate the thyroid gland and can promote the conversion of inactive thyroid hormones into their active form. While using guggul, I noticed a gradual improvement in my energy levels and metabolism. These herbs not only added a natural, holistic dimension to my wellness routine but also allowed me to connect with ancient healing traditions that have stood the test of time.

Step 5: Establish a Healthy Sleep Routine

Importance of Sleep for Thyroid Health

Sleep plays an essential role in hormone regulation, including the production and balance of thyroid hormones. For individuals managing hypothyroidism or other thyroid conditions, poor sleep can exacerbate symptoms like fatigue, brain fog, and mood disturbances, which are already common in those with thyroid imbalances. Chronic sleep deprivation can even worsen thyroid dysfunction, as sleep is crucial for the body's ability to repair itself, regulate hormones, and manage stress. A lack of quality sleep disrupts the body's circadian rhythms, impacting not only thyroid function but also overall metabolic health.

For a long time, I struggled with maintaining quality sleep, and it became clear that the more I neglected my sleep, the more my thyroid symptoms seemed to worsen. I experienced more sluggishness, difficulty concentrating, and irritability. Recognizing the link between sleep and thyroid health pushed me to prioritize my sleep routine. Making a few adjustments to my bedtime habits transformed how I felt the next day, allowing my body to reset and heal during the night.

Tips for Better Sleep

Maintain a Consistent Sleep Schedule

One of the most effective ways to improve sleep quality is by maintaining a consistent sleep schedule. Going to bed and waking up at the same time each day helps regulate your body's internal clock, or circadian rhythm. This routine allows your body to naturally synchronize its sleep-wake cycles, improving overall sleep efficiency and quality. Disrupting this rhythm, such as staying up late on weekends or frequently changing your sleep schedule, can make it harder to fall asleep and lead to more restless nights.

When I began sticking to a regular sleep schedule, it made a significant difference in how quickly I fell asleep and how rested I felt upon waking. Initially, it was difficult to maintain the same wake-up time every morning, especially on weekends when I was tempted to sleep in. However, after a couple of weeks, I noticed that my body naturally started feeling sleepy around the same time each night. This consistency not only improved my sleep but also reduced the daytime fatigue and brain fog that had been plaguing me for months. It became clear that a predictable sleep routine was a key factor in supporting both my thyroid health and overall well-being.

Create a Relaxing Bedtime Routine

Establishing a calming bedtime routine can help signal to your body that it's time to wind down and prepare for sleep. This can involve a series of activities that promote relaxation and allow you to mentally transition from the busyness of the day to a state of rest. Common practices include reading a book, journaling, listening to soft music, or taking a warm bath. The goal is to reduce stress and quiet the mind, creating a peaceful environment that encourages restful sleep.

I found that incorporating a wind-down routine had a profound impact on how easily I could fall asleep. My evenings often felt rushed, moving from one task to another, which left me feeling wired by the time I climbed into bed. By consciously setting aside time to engage in relaxing activities, I allowed my body and mind to slow down. A warm bath with Epsom salts became my favorite part of the evening, soothing both my muscles and nerves. I would follow that with some light reading or meditation, helping to clear my thoughts and relax my mind. Creating this nightly ritual not only helped improve my sleep but also contributed to a sense of balance in my life, promoting a healthier thyroid and more consistent energy levels during the day.

Limit Screen Time Before Bed

Reducing exposure to blue light from screens at least an hour before bed is another crucial step toward improving sleep quality. Devices such as phones, tablets, and computers emit blue light, which can interfere with the body's production of melatonin, the hormone that signals to the brain that it's time to sleep. Excessive blue light exposure can delay sleep onset, making it harder to fall asleep and reducing overall sleep quality. Additionally, the mental stimulation from scrolling through social media or responding to emails can prevent the mind from fully relaxing.

I realized that my habit of checking emails or scrolling through social media late into the night was contributing to my restlessness. Even after putting my phone down, I found it difficult to switch off mentally, as my mind was still processing information. When I made the decision to cut back on screen time before bed, I noticed an immediate difference in how quickly I could fall asleep. I replaced screen time with other activities like reading a physical book or engaging in light stretches, which allowed my brain to wind down naturally. Over time, limiting my screen exposure became a crucial part of my sleep routine, helping me to fall asleep faster and wake up feeling more refreshed. This simple habit improved my sleep and, as a result, helped reduce my thyroid-related symptoms like fatigue and brain fog.

By prioritizing quality sleep and incorporating these habits into my daily routine, I not only felt more rested but also saw an improvement in my thyroid health. Better sleep allowed my body to recover more efficiently, reduced stress, and improved my ability to manage daily tasks with a clearer mind. These changes have been essential in supporting my overall health, allowing me to function at my best while managing hypothyroidism.

Conclusion

A Holistic Approach to Managing Hypothyroidism

Managing hypothyroidism is far more than just taking medication; it requires a holistic approach that touches on multiple aspects of life, including diet, exercise, stress management, supplementation, and quality sleep. By focusing on these areas, individuals with hypothyroidism can significantly improve their thyroid health, reduce symptoms, and ultimately enhance their overall well-being. Every person's experience with hypothyroidism is unique, and while the following strategies may offer benefits, it's crucial to work closely with healthcare professionals to tailor an approach that suits individual needs.

Diet: Fueling Thyroid Function and Overall Health

A nutrient-rich diet is one of the cornerstones of thyroid health. Focusing on foods that support thyroid function, such as those rich in iodine, selenium, zinc, and omega-3 fatty acids, can have a profound impact on regulating thyroid hormone production and improving metabolism. Eating whole foods that provide essential vitamins and minerals allows the thyroid gland to function at its best.

For example, iodine, found in foods like seaweed, fish, and eggs, is vital for the production of thyroid hormones. Similarly, selenium, present in Brazil nuts and sunflower seeds, helps protect the thyroid from oxidative damage and supports hormone conversion. While these specific nutrients are important, a well-rounded diet that includes whole grains, lean proteins, leafy greens, and healthy fats is essential for optimal thyroid function.

Equally important is avoiding foods that could hinder thyroid function. Processed foods, loaded with unhealthy fats and sugars, can lead to inflammation and exacerbate symptoms. Likewise, certain foods like soy and raw cruciferous vegetables can interfere with thyroid hormone production when consumed excessively. By choosing fresh, whole foods over processed alternatives, and cooking goitrogenic vegetables lightly to minimize their effects, you can support your thyroid and overall health.

Exercise: Boosting Metabolism and Reducing Fatigue

Physical activity plays a pivotal role in managing hypothyroidism. Since hypothyroidism often leads to weight gain and fatigue, incorporating a regular exercise routine can help counteract these symptoms. Aerobic exercises like walking, jogging, or swimming can boost metabolism, improve cardiovascular health, and enhance energy levels. Meanwhile, strength training is essential for building muscle mass, which can increase resting metabolic rate and improve body composition.

Beyond physical health, exercise also has psychological benefits. It can lift your mood, reduce stress, and help combat the mental fatigue that often accompanies hypothyroidism. Even small efforts, such as walking or stretching, can make a noticeable difference. Starting slowly and gradually increasing the intensity of your workouts can help prevent overwhelm and allow your body to adjust to the demands of regular exercise. Flexibility exercises, such as yoga or stretching, not only help with physical well-being but also promote relaxation and stress reduction, which are crucial for individuals with hypothyroidism.

Stress Management: Calming the Mind and Supporting Thyroid Health

Chronic stress can have a significant negative impact on thyroid health. When stress levels are high, the body releases cortisol, a hormone that can inhibit the conversion of T4 (inactive thyroid hormone) to T3 (active thyroid hormone), leading to worsened symptoms. Therefore, managing stress is critical in managing hypothyroidism.

Techniques like yoga, meditation, and deep-breathing exercises can be incredibly effective in reducing stress and calming the mind. These practices help to lower cortisol levels and promote a sense of balance and well-being. Engaging in a consistent yoga practice not only strengthens the body but also offers mental clarity and emotional regulation.

Mindfulness can also be a powerful tool. By bringing your attention to the present moment and focusing on breathing or simply observing your thoughts without judgment, you can reduce the mental burden of stress. Incorporating these practices into your daily life, even for just a few minutes, can make a significant difference in how you handle stress, thus supporting your thyroid function and overall health.

Supplementation: Filling Nutritional Gaps for Thyroid Health

In addition to a healthy diet, certain supplements may be necessary to address nutrient deficiencies that could worsen thyroid health. For instance, Vitamin D, which is crucial for immune function and hormone regulation, is often deficient in individuals with hypothyroidism. Since Vitamin D is primarily absorbed through sunlight, those who live in colder climates or don't spend much time outdoors may need to supplement.

B Vitamins are also essential for energy metabolism and can help alleviate fatigue, a common symptom of hypothyroidism. Foods like quinoa, eggs, and leafy greens are rich in these vitamins, but supplementation can ensure you're getting enough. Zinc and omega-3 fatty acids are other key nutrients that support immune health and have anti-inflammatory properties, helping to manage thyroid-related inflammation.

Taking a whole-food multivitamin can also be beneficial to fill in any nutrient gaps that might be present in your diet. These vitamins and minerals, derived from natural sources, are more easily absorbed by the body and can contribute to better thyroid function and overall well-being.

Sleep: Restoring Energy and Supporting Hormone Regulation

Perhaps one of the most overlooked yet crucial aspects of managing hypothyroidism is ensuring quality sleep. Sleep is essential for hormone regulation, and individuals with hypothyroidism often struggle with fatigue due to poor sleep quality. Without enough rest, the body's ability to repair itself, regulate stress, and produce hormones is compromised, leading to worsened thyroid symptoms.

Creating a consistent sleep schedule, going to bed and waking up at the same time every day, helps regulate your circadian rhythms and improve overall sleep quality. Developing a relaxing bedtime routine, such as reading a book, practicing deep-breathing exercises, or taking a warm bath, can signal to your body that it's time to wind down.

Limiting screen time before bed is also essential, as the blue light emitted from phones, tablets, and computers can disrupt melatonin production, making it harder to fall asleep. By prioritizing good sleep hygiene and ensuring you're getting enough rest each night, you can support your body's ability to manage hypothyroidism more effectively.

Final Thoughts: A Path to Better Health

Managing hypothyroidism is an ongoing journey that requires attention to multiple aspects of health. It's about finding a balance that works for your body and making choices that support not just your thyroid, but your overall well-being. By adopting a holistic approach that includes a nutrient-rich diet, regular physical activity, stress reduction techniques, appropriate supplementation, and prioritizing quality sleep, you can empower yourself to take control of your thyroid health.

While these lifestyle changes can significantly improve your condition, it's essential to remember that hypothyroidism management should always be personalized. Consult with healthcare professionals, including doctors and nutritionists, who can guide you through this process, ensuring that your treatment plan is tailored to your unique needs. By being proactive and informed, you can live a healthier, more balanced life while managing hypothyroidism naturally.

Resources and References

- **Books:**
  - "The Thyroid Connection" by Amy Myers, M.D.
  - "The Complete Guide to Fasting" by Dr. Jason Fung
- **Websites:**
  - American Thyroid Association (thyroid.org)
  - National Institutes of Health (nih.gov)
- **Studies:**
  - Peer-reviewed articles on thyroid health, nutrition, and lifestyle interventions.